BLESSED
to Be
BROKEN

The Journey through Cancer

A THIRTY-ONE-DAY DAILY DEVOTIONAL

JAMIE BYRD

A Servant of the Lord

ISBN 978-1-68570-507-7 (paperback)
ISBN 978-1-68570-508-4 (digital)

Christian Faith Publishing
832 Park Avenue
Meadville, PA 16335
www.christianfaithpublishing.com

Printed in the United States of America

To the King eternal, immortal, invisible, the only God, and Jesus Christ, my Lord and Savior. To You, Lord, Father, Son, and Holy Spirit, be all honor and glory forever and ever. Amen!

I know that you can do all things; no purpose of yours can be thwarted.

My ears had heard of you but now my eyes have seen you. (Job 42:2, 5 NIV)

ACKNOWLEDGMENTS

Special thanks to my wife who, by her living example of faith, inspires me daily to grow closer to God; to my parents who gave me my faith as an acorn and raised me in the church to grow my faith into a mighty oak; to my mother-in-law, my second mom, who faithfully combed through this work to assure that it will be all that God has intended it to be. I love you all, and thank God for you every day.

INTRODUCTION

**My soul is weary with sorrow; strengthen
me according to your Word.**

—Psalm 119:28 NIV

**Whoever dwells in the shelter of the Most
High will rest in the shadow of the Almighty.**

—Psalm 91:1 NIV

I know a man who died on a Friday. It seemed to be a tragic death. He was a very young man. He was special, a man like the world has never seen. Many loved him, and when he died, they were disheartened and depressed. He was the glue that held his friends together. He changed their lives. Then he rose from the dead on Sunday, and the world has never been the same! What seemed like tragedy was really triumph! This is the way our Lord works in our world. Do you know this man?

I consider that our present sufferings are not worth comparing with the glory that will be revealed in us. (Romans 8:18 NIV)

The big "C" is not cancer, it's Christ! (Pat Robertson, CBN)

No one wants to have cancer or any other serious disease. But unfortunately, we don't get to choose. God allows trouble in our lives to show us how strong He is in the midst of it all and to strengthen us. It is in the midst of our troubles that we come to realize the incredible goodness and faithfulness of our Savior. If God is for us, who can be against us? (Romans 8:31)

I did not choose to have cancer, and it is important to understand that God does not generally give people cancer or any other serious disease. But our wonderful, loving God does offer comfort and peace and strength to get you through your illness. You just have to choose to receive it! **Lean into** the God of all comfort! Rest in the shadow of His wings! God's promises are for "whoever," and that includes you! Rest in the shadow of the Almighty!

These devotions contained in this book have been given to me by the Holy Spirit as I went through my cancer journey. As God told me months before I was diagnosed with cancer, my cancer journey is for His Glory! Yes, He allowed me to have cancer, but it is for His glory. It is by leaning into God that I have been able to find the incredible hope needed to survive. The Holy Spirit buoyed me up and kept me positive. If you lean into Him, get to know Him, and seek Him, He will do the same for you.

As you work through this book of devotions, meditate on God's Word. Pray, use the **journal and prayer** space after each devotion to write out your thoughts and prayers and experiences. If you need more space than is provided, add a loose leaf of paper to that page. Grow in your relationship to God through Jesus Christ, our Lord!

As you begin the journey that is ahead of you, ask your Christian friends to pray for you. Set a time each day to read the devotion and pray. Attend your church, or if you don't have one, find a church to attend which teaches the Holy Bible, to worship God, and to live among fellow believers. Iron sharpens iron! (Proverbs 27:17). I promise you that if you lean into our Savior as you fight this epic battle of life, you will be blessed in surprising ways. For by His stripes, we are healed! (Isaiah 53:5).

Yet it was the Lord's will to crush him and cause him to suffer, and though the Lord makes his

**life an offering for sin, he will see his offspring
and prolong his days, and the will of the Lord
will prosper in his hand. (Isaiah 53:10 NIV)**

God did not crucify Jesus, man did. But God allowed it to fulfill his good, divine will to save mankind. If God has allowed cancer in your life, it is for His good purpose. He is working within you. Maybe you do not belong to Him, and He wants you to be His. If you have already accepted Christ, maybe He wants you to grow closer to Him. Maybe He has some special work for you to do. Is the will of the Lord prospering in your hands? The purpose of the battle is to get you to the blessing.

You will get through this. It may be hard, but with God's help, you will get through this! Before you know it, you will be on the other side, which is a place of blessing and celebration. Just take it one day at a time. Always remember that God is in your today, and He is already in your tomorrow.

Now, may the God of all comfort and the Savior of all mankind bless you, heal you, keep you, and give you peace as only He can give! All glory and honor are yours, Almighty Father, now and forevermore!

Praise to the God of All Comfort

**Praise be to the God and Father of our Lord Jesus
Christ, the Father of compassion and the God of
all comfort, who comforts us in all our troubles,
so that we can comfort those in any trouble with
the comfort we ourselves receive from God. For
just as we share abundantly in the sufferings of
Christ, so also our comfort abounds through
Christ. (2 Corinthians 1:3–5 NIV)**

May your comfort abound through Christ! **Amen!**

But let all who take refuge in you be glad; let them ever sing for joy. Spread your protection over them, that those who love your name may rejoice in you. Surely, LORD, you bless the righteous; you surround them with your favor as with a shield. (Psalm 5:11–12 NIV)

It was good for me to be afflicted so that I might learn your decrees. (Psalm 119:71 NIV)

Overhearing what they said, Jesus told him, "Don't be afraid; just believe." (Mark 5:36 NIV)

Blessed are the pure in heart, for they will see God. (Matthew 5:8 NIV)

My sacrifice, O God, is a broken spirit; a broken and contrite heart you, God, will not despise. (Psalm 51:17 NIV)

Lift up your eyes and look to the heavens: Who created all these? He who brings out the starry host one by one and calls forth each of them by name. Because of his great power and mighty strength, not one of them is missing.

Why do you complain, Jacob? Why do you say, Israel, "My way is hidden from the Lord; my cause is disregarded by my God"?

Do you not know? Have you not heard? The Lord is the everlasting God, the Creator of the ends of the earth. He will not grow tired or weary, and his understanding no one can fathom.

He gives strength to the weary and increases the power of the weak. Even youths grow tired and weary, and young men stumble and fall; but those who hope in the Lord will renew their strength. They will soar on wings like eagles; they will run and not grow weary, they will walk and not be faint. (Isaiah 40:26– 31 NIV)

Journal and Prayer

PAGE OF FAITH

Add your own survivors to the list! At the writing of this book:

- Pastor David Jeremiah had stage IV lymphoma twenty-five years ago and still enjoys his full life.
- My sister had metastatic breast cancer six years ago and continues to have no recurrence.
- My father had colon cancer ten years ago and is doing well with no recurrence.
- My sister-in-law had Non-Hodgkin's lymphoma thirty years ago and has had no recurrence.
- Dodie Osteen, Joel Osteen's mother, has survived terminal liver cancer for forty years.

DAY ONE

**Just as the Son of Man did not come
to be served, but to serve, and to give
his life as a ransom for many.**

—Matthew 20:28 NIV

A few weeks ago, while I was visiting my parents, I noticed a lump in my neck. After having it CT-scanned, my doctor told me that it was abnormal and needed to be biopsied to see if it was cancer.

I have lived long enough now to have been in many bad circumstances. I know all too well the feelings of dread and despair that often accompany bad news. It is really tempting to cry out to God, "This is not fair!" But God wants a different response from us. You see, our response to the events in our life becomes our life story. What do you want your life story to be? More importantly, what does God want your life story to be? Just as Jesus came to serve, this is what we are called to do.

John 8:12 (NIV) says,

When Jesus spoke again to the people, He said, "I am the light of the world. Whoever follows me will never walk in darkness but will have the light of life."

1

Despite the darkness, despite the possibility for bad news, I chose to focus on the Light. I recognize that whatever part of my story this is, whether the middle or the end, I will trust God. I can see that, whatever this is, God is allowing it for His Glory and my good. I recognize fully and completely that to live is Christ and to die is gain. And I trust God completely with the outcome.

As a result, I have no fear. I have no dread. I am not worried about this lump and its implications. I have given it to God and seek only to glorify His name and to serve. All glory, honor, and praise to God, the Father, and to Jesus Christ, His Son and my Savior. I have entered the rest of God!

So what about you? You can also enjoy God's strength and power. You can also receive His peace.

Psalm 31:1–5 (NIV), a psalm of David, says,

> **In you, Lord, I have taken refuge; let me never be put to shame; deliver me in your righteousness.**
>
> **Turn your ear to me, come quickly to my rescue; be my rock of refuge, a strong fortress to save me.**
>
> **Since you are my rock and my fortress, for the sake of your name lead and guide me.**
>
> **Keep me free from the trap that is set for me, for you are my refuge.**
>
> **Into your hands I commit my spirit; deliver me, Lord, my faithful God.**

> **When He heard this, Jesus said, "This sickness will not end in death. No, it is for God's glory so that God's Son may be glorified through it." (John 11:4 NIV)**

> **For to me, to live is Christ and to die is gain. (Philippians 1:21 NIV)**

Though He slay me, yet will I trust Him. (Job 13:15 NKJV)

If this cancer takes my life one day, do not say, "He lost his battle with cancer." Instead, say, "He won his battle in life, and he is with his Savior in victory!" This is the truth of my life! This, too, can be the truth in yours! If you somehow understand why you have cancer, it will not provide you with any peace and will not provide you with any joy. So trying to figure out why is a waste of time. But knowing and trusting in the goodness and faithfulness of our incredible, loving God can give you peace and joy.

**I know that my redeemer lives, and that
in the end He will stand on the earth.
And after my skin has been destroyed,
yet in my flesh I will see God;
I myself will see him with my own
eyes—I, and not another. How
my heart yearns within me!**

—Job 19:25–27 NIV

Journal and Prayer

DAY TWO

**You will keep in perfect peace those whose
minds are steadfast, because they trust in you.**

—Isaiah 26:3 NIV

Last week, I found out that I have cancer. As you know or would imagine, the moment someone tells you something like this is unforgettable. But I was not afraid. I did not feel sorry for myself. I wasn't worried. I did not take on a feeling of dread. I just leaned into my all-powerful Savior. I handed this diagnosis to Him and placed my trust in God!

A few months ago, in my daily prayer life with God, He revealed to me that I was going to have cancer. But He said that my having cancer would be for His glory. I said, "Yes, Lord. I will obey!" You see, I trust my God! I trust Him enough to be able to face cancer without being afraid. You can trust God to get you through this.

Years ago, God gave me a verse to be my life verse:

> **Trust in the Lord with all your heart and lean
> not on your own understanding; in all your
> ways submit to him, and He will make your
> paths straight. (Proverbs 3:5–6 NIV)**

When He gave me that verse, I was not there yet. I was still learning to trust the Lord. But He lovingly showed me the way. The great potter molded me and shaped me into the man He wanted me to be. He wanted a disciple of Christ! I submitted myself to His way.

I could not become this man on my own. It is only in submitting to God and in trusting him that we become the person that He wants us to be. But when you choose to submit to Him, He comes to live in you. We rest in the shadow of His wings!

God did not give me this cancer. He allowed it, but He did not give it to me. All things pass through God's hands—good and bad. But He is the God who turns all things to good (Romans 8:28). I know that there will be a day, just as there's a day for all of us, that I will die. But that day will not be today, and it will not be tomorrow. That day will be the day that the Lord has decided. **It has never been any other way.** And that day will not happen until the Lord is through with me here. So I will serve the Lord until that day comes. I will serve the Lord until He calls me home. And what a glorious day that will be!

When you learn to completely trust in God, you receive the power and faithfulness of our Almighty Creator. Yes, you rest in the shadow of His wings. You can face daunting challenges in faith. Our God is the God who takes us **through** the valley of the shadow of death (Psalm 23). He is the God who is bigger than any problem, sickness, and diagnosis. He is the same God who created our world and everything around us. He can squash cancer just as easily as we can wet our fingers and put out a candle. He is ALMIGHTY GOD! Whether He does or not is not a matter of my concern. I trust Him! I am here to do His will!

Worry is the product of not trusting God. You cannot place your trust in money. You cannot put your trust in good health. You cannot put your trust in your family. You cannot put your trust in your church. You cannot put your trust in your career. These parts of your life are capable of letting you down. Your worry about these things is full evidence that they will let you down. God is the only one whom you can trust. He will never leave you nor forsake you!

So give it all to Him! Give Him your finances, and ask Him before spending your money. Give Him your health; indeed give Him your life that He may spend it in the right way. Give Him your family. Give Him your marriage. Give Him your children even before they are born. Give Him your church, and let Him lead you to the right place where your faith can grow. Give Him your career that you may work diligently for the Lord *at whatever you do*, and bring Him glory! And most of all, pray fervently for this. Keep your eye on the face of God! He will make your path straight!

This cancer is not my burden. Just as everything I am, belongs to God through Christ Jesus, this cancer, too, belongs to God. Although He allowed it, He did not give it to me. Having placed it in His care, why should I take it away from Him? I will not! There is no better place for every aspect of our life to be than in the hands of God! I trust Him to make my path straight. I even trust Him to make this into something for good. May God be praised! For the Lord inhabits the praises of His people! (Psalm 22:3).

It is not uncommon to hear people say that God will not give you more than you can bear. After all, this is in the Bible. However, I would alter this statement slightly. God does not give you bad things in your life. These things come from the world, from the evil one, or from our own bad choices. I would say that God will never allow you to have more than you can bear **with Him.** On your own, you are sunk. But all things are possible with God! And it is in Him and through Him that you can make it through. It doesn't matter what is happening in your world. What matters is your relationship with God. This is where you will find enough power to have peace! Our God is bigger than whatever you may face. Jesus told us,

> **I have told you these things, so that in me you may have peace. In this world you will have trouble. But take heart! I have overcome the world. (John 16:33 NIV)**

All glory and honor are yours Almighty God, now and forevermore! Come, Lord Jesus! I praise your Holy name! Amen!

———————————

Journal and Prayer

DAY THREE

**I remain confident of this: I will see the
goodness of the Lord in the land of the living.**

—Psalm 27:13 NIV

For years, I have put scriptures on my mirror so that I would see them every time I went into my bathroom. They help me stay focused in the right direction and give me encouragement often when I need it most.

When I found out that I had cancer, I knew that I was going to need more encouragement. And our ever-faithful God provided me with what I needed. Years ago, as mentioned in the previous devotion, God gave me a scripture that has become my life scripture. It is Proverbs 3:5–6, which I have memorized and frequently quote:

> **Trust in the Lord with all your heart and lean
> not on your own understanding; in all your
> ways submit to him, and He will make your
> paths straight. (Proverbs 3:5–6 NIV)**

This scripture has been a light unto my path. When I have been facing trials, this scripture has helped me find my way.

As I was praying about my journey with cancer and preparing myself for the battle, God gave me the next two verses:

Do not be wise in your own eyes; fear the Lord and shun evil.

This will bring health to your body and nourishment to your bones. (Proverbs 3:7–8 NIV)

It's funny, but although I have read those verses many times, they did not speak to me until the Holy Spirit pointed them out to me. I found additional strength and encouragement in the Word of the Lord! In my spirit, I could hear the Lord telling me,

Don't let the battles in your life become bigger than the God you serve!

God is moving through you! He is with you and for you! Rest in the shadow of His wings, for He is your fortress and refuge! The test you face now will become your testimony! You can count on God to be with you! We can absolutely have faith in our living God! Don't allow yourself to think this battle is bigger than God. It is not! God is well able to get you through this if you will lean into Him and trust Him. Give this battle to the Lord, and you will be blessed!

But the Lord has become my fortress, and my God the rock in whom I take refuge.

—Psalm 94:22 NIV

Journal and Prayer

Day Four

**Do not be anxious about anything, but
in every situation, by prayer and petition,
with thanksgiving, present your requests
to God. And the peace of God, which
transcends all understanding, will guard
your hearts and your minds in Christ Jesus.**

—Philippians 4:6–7 NIV

Whenever you find yourself worrying, it means you should be praying. The Bible tells us that we should not worry (Matthew 6:25–34). Worry robs you of the good life that God has planned for you.

Therefore do not worry about tomorrow, for tomorrow will worry about itself. Each day has enough trouble of its own. (Matthew 6:34)

Prayer, on the other hand, is conversation with God:

The Prayer of Faith

Is anyone among you in trouble? Let them pray. Is anyone happy? Let them sing songs of praise. Is anyone among you sick? Let them

10

> **call the elders of the church to pray over them
> and anoint them with oil in the name of the
> Lord. And the prayer offered in faith will make
> the sick person well; the Lord will raise them
> up. If they have sinned, they will be forgiven.
> (James 5:13–15 NIV)**

Begin by recognizing and acknowledging who God is and His sovereignty over all things. Confess your sins, including your worry, and ask for forgiveness. Thank Him for being active in your life, for loving you, for giving you His Spirit to guide you, and for Jesus to save you. Thank Him for the many blessings in your life. Then present your request to God.

And if you are married, you should pray every week with your spouse. If you are not married, find a relative or friend or pastor who will pray with you. There is power when you pray with another believer in Jesus's name! Jesus tells us this Himself in Matthew:

> **"Truly I tell you, whatever you bind on earth
> will be bound in heaven, and whatever you
> loose on earth will be loosed in heaven.**
>
> **"Again, truly I tell you that if two of you
> on earth agree about anything they ask for, it
> will be done for them by my Father in heaven.
> For where two or three gather in my name,
> there am I with them." (Matthew 18:18–20
> NIV)**

Praying with someone else can sometimes seem awkward at first for some people. Talk with your prayer partner about the power of praying together and what you want to pray about. Remember what comes with praying together: peace, guarded hearts and minds, and answered prayers.

Gather in Jesus's name. He will come to meet you in your storm! He has promised that He will be with you. He says, "For where two or three gather in my name, there am I with them." He will hear your prayer and intercede. He will get you through this!

**Heal me, Lord, and I will be healed;
save me and I will be saved, for
you are the one I praise.**

—Jeremiah 17:14 (NIV)

**Ask me, and I will make the
nations your inheritance, the ends
of the earth your possession.**

—Psalm 2:8 (NIV)

———————

Journal and Prayer

DAY FIVE

**Jesus answered, "I am the way and the truth
and the life. No one comes to the Father
except through me. If you really know me,
you will know my Father as well. From now
on, you do know him and have seen him."**

—John 14:6–7 (NIV)

The home I live in, the car I drive each day, the things I enjoy in my life, even my wife and family, do not really belong to me. With the cancer I am fighting, it is possible that I will die from it. But regardless of whether you have cancer or not, the probability of death for each one of us is 100 percent. There's no one who can escape it!

So having considered this, it is impossible not to realize that God is the only aspect of our lives that transcends death. He is really all that we have—nothing else really matters! And if you have not accepted Christ, and you do not have God in your life, then really you have nothing.

Can you be happy with God alone in your life? You can if you seek His face and come to know Him. Come to experience the incredible love of the Father through the Son, Jesus Christ! Don't wait to discover that He is all you need until He is all you have.

There is comfort in knowing that you have been saved by the blood of Jesus Christ. More than that, there is a power in knowing that you have been saved by the blood of Jesus Christ. Houses crumble, cars fail, eventually, everyone you know will die. So the greatest hope that you can have is found in our Savior, Jesus Christ. It is only through Christ that you can have eternal life. So even if this cancer takes my life, to live is to serve Christ, and to die is to be with Christ! (Philippians 1:21).

In **My Utmost for His Highest**, Oswald Chambers wrote,

> The experience the psalmist speaks of—"We will not fear, even though…" (Psalm 46:2)—will be ours once we are grounded on the truth of the reality of God's presence, not just a simple awareness of it, but an understanding of the reality of it. (Utmost.org, July 20)

As I prepare to begin my treatment, I can feel the presence of the Holy Spirit with me. His power fills me and reminds me that I am not alone. I am wrapped in the loving arms of God! I am fully depending on God, and there is no better place to be. This is available to each and every child of God! It is received by becoming a disciple of Christ.

Anxiety is imagining a future without God's presence. God will be with you in your future! Just as God gave the Israelites manna from heaven and only for a day, God gives His grace to you day by day. And as a disciple of Christ, you always have enough grace to face whatever comes your way with God. Whatever you may be facing, you can face it fearlessly with God. The path to this is found in accepting Jesus Christ as your Savior and spending daily time with our wonderful Lord. He is the way, the truth, and the life! (John 14:6).

Come to me, all you who are weary and burdened, and I will give you rest. Take my yoke upon you and learn from me, for I am gentle and humble in heart, and

**you will find rest for your souls. For my
yoke is easy and my burden is light.**

—Matthew 11:28–30 (NIV)

Journal and Prayer

Day Six

Jesus Predicts His Death

**From that time on Jesus began to explain to
his disciples that He must go to Jerusalem
and suffer many things at the hands of the
elders, the chief priests and the teachers
of the law, and that He must be killed
and on the third day be raised to life.**

**Peter took him aside and began to
rebuke him. "Never, Lord!" He said.
"This shall never happen to you!"**

**Jesus turned and said to Peter, "Get behind
me, Satan! You are a stumbling block to
me; you do not have in mind the concerns
of God, but merely human concerns."**

—Matthew 16:21–23 (NIV)

Ever since I found out that I have cancer, I have never felt sorry
for myself. Yes, it has been hard. There has been pain and suffering.
But I have never felt sorry for myself. Instead, the Holy Spirit has
reminded me that our God is the one who makes all things work

together for our good (Romans 8:28)—even cancer. So you should not feel sorry for yourself or elicit feelings of sympathy from others. Instead, set your face like a flint to find and expect the goodness of the Lord! (Isaiah 50:7).

Jesus sets the example for us in today's scripture reading. Peter, filled with his love for his friend and master, acts only out of his feelings in defiance to God's will for Jesus. He wasn't intentionally defying God, but He could not yet see the incredible goodness at the core of God's plan for Jesus: salvation for mankind. We can learn from this.

Instead of giving into human emotion, embrace the incredible hope that we have in Christ to transcend this life and live one day in cancer-free bodies (Philippians 3:20–21). Pray for insight and assistance from God in finding your way (James 1:5). Ask others to pray for this for you (James 5:16). Fill your mind with God's promises through reading Scripture (Colossians 3:2, Daniel 10:12). Embrace the promise that God can make all things—anything— work together for your good (Romans 8:28). And wait patiently with expectation for the good that God has planned for you (Psalm 27:14, Psalm 37:7). He has already planned it (Philippians 4:19). You just have to expect it and wait for the appointed time (Psalm 5:3). It's on the way!

Finally, whenever the evil one tries to make you feel sorry for yourself, remind yourself that we are children of the most high God. He has promised you goodness! You can do all things through Christ, who gives you strength! (Philippians 4:13) And crush that evil one under your feet! (Genesis 3:15).

I remain confident of this: I will see the goodness of the Lord in the land of the living.

—Psalm 27:13 NIV

Now to him who is able to do immeasurably more than all we ask or imagine, according to his power that is at work

**within us, to him be glory in the church
and in Christ Jesus throughout all
generations, for ever and ever! Amen.**

—**Ephesians 3:20–21 NIV**

Further study: also see Romans 8 and 12.

_____

Journal and Prayer

DAY SEVEN

**Therefore, in order to keep me from
becoming conceited, I was given a thorn in
my flesh, a messenger of Satan, to torment
me. Three times I pleaded with the Lord
to take it away from me. But he said to
me, "My grace is sufficient for you, for
my power is made perfect in weakness."
Therefore I will boast all the more gladly
about my weaknesses, so that Christ's power
may rest on me. That is why, for Christ's
sake, I delight in weaknesses, in insults, in
hardships, in persecutions, in difficulties.
For when I am weak, then I am strong.**

—2 Corinthians 12:7–10

I have discovered that when you get cancer, it doesn't just invade
your body; it also invades your mind and soul. Cancer invades your
finances and relationships. Indeed, it invades your faith. It really is an
insidious disease! So how do you survive this?

The truth is that even with the pain from the chemo and the
radiation treatments, the cancer in my body has been nothing com-
pared to what seems like cancer for the rest of my life. Occasionally,
I have trouble sleeping. But it's not the cancer in my body that is

keeping me awake. It's the cancer in my home that is found in my leaky roof and in an expensive new air conditioner that won't work properly. It's the cancer in my personal finances that were caused by the cancer that killed my career long before I even got sick.

I have prayed for years for relief, but no relief has come. It seems that every step that I take to improve my situation ends up in a cancerous dead end with no sign of improvement and nowhere to go. At times, I've become so disheartened that I can hardly pray anymore. Have I lived too long with no answer and relief? Can my faith survive this? How do I figure out where to go from here?

Have you ever felt this way? Yes, sometimes life can be this way, life can give you thorns, but it has not been wasted. This pattern in my life has helped me to become the person God wants me to be. Do not allow the darkness to overcome you. In fact, for me, this is a path to my sanctification and to becoming the man God wants me to be.

Do you not know that your bodies are temples of the Holy Spirit, who is in you, whom you have received from God? You are not your own. (1 Corinthians 6:19 NIV)

These troubles have molded me. They have humbled me and sharpened my focus. They have helped me submit to the Lord. They have equipped me for God's work. The Lord will provide for all your needs just as He has for me.

The Sovereign Lord has given me a well-instructed tongue, to know the word that sustains the weary. He wakens me morning by morning, wakens my ear to listen like one being instructed.

The Sovereign Lord has opened my ears; I have not been rebellious, I have not turned away.

I offered my back to those who beat me, my cheeks to those who pulled out my beard;

I did not hide my face from mocking and spitting.

Because the Sovereign Lord helps me, I will not be disgraced. Therefore have I set my face like flint, and I know I will not be put to shame. (Isaiah 50:4–7 NIV)

You should not fear what seems like darkness, for you are **hidden in the shadow of the Lord's hand**. This is your calling. This is your inheritance. This cancer is part of your journey. Believe it or not, it is leading you to your **source of strength and power** in Jesus Christ. It is for your sanctification. It is for your good. Like fire that burns the dross off of gold or silver to make it pure, this part of your life is purifying you. Set your face like a flint to get through it. This battle will be won on your knees and by leaning into your Savior. Lean into and be strong in the Lord! He is worthy of your trust and faith! Lean and be strong in the Lord! He is doing amazing work in you, and it is all for your good.

In his letter to the Philippians, the Apostle Paul wrote,

I know how to be abased and live humbly in straitened circumstances, and I know also how to enjoy plenty and live in abundance. I have learned in any and all circumstances the secret of facing every situation, whether well-fed or going hungry, having a sufficiency and enough to spare or going without and being in want.

I have strength for all things in Christ Who empowers me [I am ready for anything and equal to anything through Him Who infuses inner strength into me; I am self-sufficient in Christ's sufficiency]. (Philippians 4:12–13 AMPC)

You **can do** all things through Christ, who strengthens you! Fix your eyes on Him. God makes you strong in your weakness. When you feel weak, you are strong!

> **The stone the builders rejected has become the cornerstone; the Lord has done this, and it is marvelous in our eyes. The Lord has done it this very day; let us rejoice today and be glad.**
>
> **—Psalm 118:22–24 NIV**

God provided funding for my new roof and led me to a new AC service who could properly repair my air conditioning unit. He will meet all my needs. He will meet all of your needs too.

Journal and Prayer

DAY EIGHT

The Parable of the Lost Son

Jesus continued: "There was a man who had two sons. The younger one said to his father, 'Father, give me my share of the estate.' So he divided his property between them.

"Not long after that, the younger son got together all he had, set off for a distant country and there squandered his wealth in wild living. After he had spent everything, there was a severe famine in that whole country, and he began to be in need. So he went and hired himself out to a citizen of that country, who sent him to his fields to feed pigs. *16* He longed to fill his stomach with the pods that the pigs were eating, but no one gave him anything.

"When he came to his senses, he said, 'How many of my father's hired servants have food to spare, and here I am starving to death! I will set out and go back to my father and say to him: Father, I have sinned against heaven and against you. I am no longer worthy to be called your son; make me like one of your hired servants.' So he got up and went to his father.

"But while he was still a long way off, his father saw him and was filled with compassion for him; he ran to his son, threw his arms around him and kissed him.

"The son said to him, 'Father, I have sinned against heaven and against you. I am no longer worthy to be called your son.'

"But the father said to his servants, 'Quick! Bring the best robe and put it on him. Put a ring on his finger and sandals on his feet. Bring the fattened calf and kill it. Let's have a feast and celebrate. For this son of mine was dead and is alive again; he was lost and is found.' So, they began to celebrate.

—Luke 15:11–24 NIV

You may be wealthier than you think! It seems I get an envelope in my mailbox about once a month with this statement on the outside. I always thought it was just some come-on from an advertiser trying to get me to consider them for wealth management. And so I have always ignored the messages, even scoffing at them as I throw them in the trash—until the Holy Spirit whispered in my ear, "You may be wealthier than you think!"

The Spirit convicted me and pointed out the statements I have made:

- "I will never be able to retire."
- "I will never be able to make enough money to pay all my bills."
- "I will never be able to live my life completely for God because I'm going to have to always work at some job to pay the bills."

I did not just make these complaints directly to God in my prayers, but as I made these statements in my home out loud, I created a self-fulfilling prophecy for myself. More than that, I allowed the devil to fill my thoughts with his lies and trained myself to believe them. Once I realized this, or I should say that once the Holy Spirit pointed this out to me, I immediately prayed and asked God to forgive me.

You see, you and I who have accepted Christ as our Savior are adopted sons and daughters of the Creator of the universe. We are the children of Almighty God who owns **all things**, even those things like our home and our car that we are under the illusion that we own. We are all lost sons and daughters.

As I prayed, I also asked God to change my thinking, to lead me to the understanding that He wants me to have about money and wealth, and to lead my every step and choice as I make decisions concerning my life moving forward. I don't know for sure, but I think He is pleased that I'm finally listening to Him about this. I also think He will be glad to no longer hear my complaints about this.

One of my pastor friends likes to say that our God owns a thousand cattle on a thousand hills (Psalm 50). He has said it many times in my presence in the last year. The Lord is gently persistent! I'm so grateful to our God for His loving persistence!

So this is a new perspective for me! I feel completely free from the lies from the devil about my personal finances. I can see the future that God has prepared for me, and it gives me great hope! I am excited about learning the ways of God's economy instead of trying to muddle my way along in the world's economy. God's economy is an economy of blessing.

> **And my God shall supply all your need according to His riches in glory by Christ Jesus. (Philippians 4:19 NKJV)**

Now, what about you?

When the lost son came home, he was given a fine robe symbolizing his father's forgiveness of all that he has done—the robe of righteousness. He was given a ring for his finger to symbolize the father's restoration of authority to him as a son. And he was given shoes for his feet, symbolizing the restoration of his rights as a son. You see, the father has always loved the son. He has never stopped. In the son's eyes, the father loved him far more than he deserved.

Our Father has always loved you, and He has never stopped. Jesus told this parable for me. Jesus told this parable for you. Isn't it time to really work at becoming one with Christ and one with the Father? Isn't it time to finally get on board with all that our Father wants to do in your life? Our Father is waiting with your robe in His hands.

———————

Journal and Prayer

DAY NINE

**The righteous person may have
many troubles, but the Lord
delivers him from them all;**

—Psalm 34:19 NIV

My radiation treatments have left me with dead taste buds. I can no longer enjoy food. And my chemo treatments have left me sick and nauseated for days. Trouble seems to be an integral part of having cancer as well as life itself. But that's not all there is. I wonder if you see the rest of it?

There are blessings too. I have a lot more time to spend in God's Word and to grow closer to God. I have more time to spend in prayer. The Holy Spirit has blessed me with new insights into God's Word and the world that we live in. I have been able to spend more time with my wife. And God has given me new work to do for Him. And there are more blessings for me to discover! What about you?

Your life can become blessed or troubled by whichever one you choose to focus on. They both exist in your life, **but do you see the blessings**? If not, do not despair. The devil is blinding you from these. He wants you to always feel bad.

The evil one spends all of his time trying to make sure that you see and focus on the troubles. But it takes effort to find the blessings that Christ is providing for you every day. This is because the evil one is working hard to keep you from seeing them. You must oppose him! Don't let him win by focusing on your troubles!

King David knew this and shared it with us in Psalm 34. During the time that he wrote this, David was facing certain death unless the Lord delivered him.

> **I will extol the Lord at all times; his praise will always be on my lips.**
>
> **I will glory in the Lord; let the afflicted hear and rejoice.**
>
> **Glorify the Lord with me; let us exalt his name together.**
>
> **I sought the Lord, and he answered me; he delivered me from all my fears.**
>
> **Those who look to him are radiant; their faces are never covered with shame.**
>
> **This poor man called, and the Lord heard him; he saved him out of all his troubles.**
>
> **The angel of the Lord encamps around those who fear him, and he delivers them.**
>
> **Taste and see that the Lord is good; blessed is the one who takes refuge in him. (Psalm 34:1–8 NIV)**

If you are not already doing so, it is time to take charge of your life and look for your blessings. If you do this, you will find joy and abundant life **no matter what else you are facing.** You may have many troubles, but the Lord can deliver you from them! He will make a way! Leave your troubles at the foot of the cross and expect good things from the Lord!

**Taste and see that the Lord is good; blessed
is the one who takes refuge in him.**

—Psalm 34:8 NIV

Further study: see Psalm 103.

_____

Journal and Prayer

DAY TEN

Moses and the Burning Bush

Now Moses was tending the flock of Jethro his father-in-law, the priest of Midian, and he led the flock to the far side of the wilderness and came to Horeb, the mountain of God. There the angel of the LORD appeared to him in flames of fire from within a bush. Moses saw that though the bush was on fire it did not burn up. So Moses thought, "I will go over and see this strange sight—why the bush does not burn up."

When the LORD saw that he had gone over to look, God called to him from within the bush, "Moses! Moses!"

And Moses said, "Here I am."

"Do not come any closer," God said. "Take off your sandals, for the place where you are standing is holy ground."

—Exodus 3:1–5 NIV

One of the comedians from my youth talked about how, if he was misbehaving, his mother would take off her shoe and hit him in the

30

head with it from across the room. As I recall, her shoe always had a boomerang action and would return to her hand after it smacked him in the head. Moms are pretty incredible people, and I believe this is possible. But I don't think she gave up any of her rights as a mom.

In ancient Israel, taking off your shoes was symbolic of giving up your rights. Every Jewish person knew this. When Moses saw the burning bush, he was told to take off his shoes. And he complied without reservation or hesitation. He gave up all of his rights to God. And God was able to use him for great purposes because he submitted. He led the Israelites out of Egypt, received the Ten Commandments from God, and wrote a significant portion of the Old Testament. Glory be to God!

If you want to really be used by God, you have to give Him your shoes. Giving your shoes to God means fully submitting to Him. It can mean giving God your career. It can mean giving God your favorite hobby. It can mean giving God your finances. It can mean giving God your reservations about the truth of the Bible. It can mean giving God more of your time. If you really like shoes, it can mean actually giving God your shoes. It can even mean all of these things. The point is that we voluntarily give up our rights in favor of serving God and doing His will. You can never do great things for God without giving Him your shoes.

Now understand, God does not demand your shoes or that you submit to Him. But in my experience, the more you know God, the more you know how wonderful He is, the more you know His grace and mercy, the more you want to give Him your shoes. Indeed, you want to give Him everything! And if you do this, it will be the greatest thing you have ever done! You see, you cannot out give God (Malachi 3:10).

So submit to God, and see what great things He has planned for you! Give Him your shoes, and be blessed!

_____

Journal and Prayer

Day Eleven

A prayer of an afflicted person who has grown weak and pours out a lament before the Lord.

Hear my prayer, Lord; let my cry for help come to you.

Do not hide your face from me when I am in distress. Turn your ear to me; when I call, answer me quickly.

For my days vanish like smoke; my bones burn like glowing embers.

My heart is blighted and withered like grass; I forget to eat my food.

In my distress I groan aloud and am reduced to skin and bones.

I am like a desert owl, like an owl among the ruins.

I lie awake; I have become like a bird alone on a roof.

All day long my enemies taunt me; those who rail against me use my name as a curse.

For I eat ashes as my food and mingle my drink with tears because of your great wrath, for you have taken me up and thrown me aside.

**My days are like the evening shadow; I
wither away like grass.**

—Psalm 102 NIV

I have been down for most of the last four days. I got really sick after my most recent chemo treatment. I have not been able to eat or even function. Unfortunately, this seems to be normal for me. I get really sick after my chemo.

After my radiation treatment yesterday, I met with my radiation oncologist. He was not pleased with how I was feeling nor with the six pounds I lost seemingly overnight. After talking with me and examining me, he worked with me to formulate a different strategy to try and overcome my feeling so bad. He told me not to wait until I felt nauseated to take my anti-nausea medicine. He said, take it as soon as I get up to get ahead of the nausea. He also gave me an additional script to try.

While I have felt bad, I have not been depressed during this time of treatment. Perhaps it's because I have prayed my way through this illness so far. I have not just been praying for myself, but I've been praying for my friends and family and people I know who really need prayer right now—even my enemies. I believe we are blessed by what God passes through us. So when we pray fervently for others, we also receive from the Lord.

I have not been eating because my food tastes like ashes in my mouth. Nothing tastes good. In His still, small voice, Abba led me to this scripture, Psalm 102. He comforts me in my distress. He reminds me of His love for me and that He can make all things new again. He is all-powerful, able to whip up a storm with a thought, but He is gentle enough to comfort me when I need it most—even someone as insignificant as me. I love my Abba! Thank you for choosing me to be yours, Almighty Father! He has chosen you too!

**You did not choose me, but I chose you
and appointed you so that you might go
and bear fruit—fruit that will last.**

—John 15:16 NIV

Journal and Prayer

DAY TWELVE

**He says, "Be still, and know that I
am God; I will be exalted among the
nations, I will be exalted in the earth."**

—Psalm 46:10 (NIV)

I was watching *Duck Dynasty* on television. It is so good to watch a Christian TV show! In this episode, we find out that one of the brothers has a daughter named Mia, who was born with a cleft palate. She has had several surgeries to correct the problem and was getting ready to have another one. At her request, they threw a family reunion party in her honor.

At one point, they invited her to come and speak to everyone. She quoted the scripture above, Psalm 46:10, as her favorite verse. She said it was her favorite verse because whenever she was facing any difficulty, it reminded her of how great our God is and that He is way bigger than our troubles. This is pretty impressive for a ten- or twelve-year-old girl.

The seed for this faith was given to her by the Holy Spirit and nurtured by her parents. The trials she has faced and the valleys she has walked through have grown her faith and filled her with God's strength. I wish I had such faith when I was her age. But such faith only comes by trial.

They prayed for her as a family, and when she had her surgery, the Robertson's were there with her. What a brave young lady!

You too will find new strength as you walk through this valley. God is with you, and He is upholding you with His righteous right hand!

> **So do not fear, for I am with you; do not**
> **be dismayed, for I am your God. I will**
> **strengthen you and help you; I will uphold**
> **you with my righteous right hand.**
>
> **—Isaiah 41:10 NIV**

For more information, see www.miamoo.org.

Journal and Prayer

And so we know and rely on the love God has for us. God is love. Whoever lives in love lives in God, and God in them. (1 John 4:16 NIV)

Hear, O Israel: The Lord our God, the Lord is one. Love the Lord your God with all your heart and with all your soul and with all your strength. These commandments that I give you today are to be on your hearts. Impress them on your children. Talk about them when you sit at home and when you walk along the road, when you lie down and when you get up. Tie them as symbols on your hands and bind them on your foreheads. Write them on the doorframes of your houses and on your gates. (Deuteronomy 6:4–9 NIV)

Whatever you do, work at it with all your heart, as working for the Lord, not for human masters, since you know that you will receive an inheritance from the Lord as a reward. It is the Lord Christ you are serving. (Colossians 3:23–24 NIV)

Journal and Prayer

DAY THIRTEEN

**Sanctify them by the truth;
your Word is truth.**

—John 17:17 (NIV)

This is an important lesson for all of us to learn. The world wants you to believe that **what you feel** is truth. What you feel is real, but it is not truth. When people begin to believe that their feelings are truth, it leads to strife and dissension. It leads to bad choices and mistakes. Mistaking feelings for truth pushes people apart because everyone has a different truth.

The scripture above comes from Jesus's prayer for His disciples just before He was going to the cross. He prays that we will be sanctified in the truth. Then He points out that God's Word is the truth.

Jesus is the way, the truth, and the life (John 14:6). There is no other truth. Everything else is just opinion. But don't take my word for it. Take the word of Jesus Christ!

It might be tempting to think, "That is a pretty exclusive way to think!" After all, there are many people who do not believe in Jesus Christ as Lord and Savior. But actually, it is a very inclusive way to think.

**For God so loved the world that he gave his
one and only Son, that whoever believes in**

**him shall not perish but have eternal life.
(John 3:16 NIV)**

You see, God gave His son for **whoever believes**. That **whoever** means anyone! God gives us the choice! He doesn't forcibly make you believe but instead invites you to receive His gift of salvation. **Whoever** means everyone and anyone is invited. The only way you will not be included is if you **choose** not to be and do not accept Christ as your savior. As the Lord says in the book of Deuteronomy, "I put before you life and death. Choose life!"

> **This day I call the heavens and the earth as witnesses against you that I have set before you life and death, blessings and curses. Now choose life, so that you and your children may live. (Deuteronomy 30:19 NIV)**

Jesus tells us in John 10:10,

> **The thief comes only to steal and kill and destroy; I have come that they may have life, and have it to the full. (John 10:10 NIV)**

To quote Walt Kelly's *Pogo* cartoon from 1971, "We have met the enemy and he is us!"

Journal and Prayer

DAY FOURTEEN

**A good name is more desirable
than great riches; to be esteemed
is better than silver or gold.**

—Proverbs 22:1 (NIV)

"Good morning, James!" James is my given name, the name of my father. It is my formal name, the official name that is on every legal document pertaining to me. And now it has become my cancer name, the name the health-care workers call me because they do not know me.

Before I got cancer, I had thought about changing my "called" name to James from Jamie to reflect the change in me brought about through Christ. Somehow, it seems appropriate to me to change the name people use to address me since I am not who I used to be before Christ. When Saul was changed by Christ, he became known as Paul. Plus, in the Bible, Jesus's half-brother, James, wrote a great book that everyone should read. It is hard to understand at first, but it is the absolute truth. Understanding comes with maturity in your relationship with Jesus. So then changing my "called" name to James has lots of merits. Despite this, I have never made a change in name. And I am okay with that. After all, the name may not have changed, but the man is very different!

So then, I have indeed become James, the disciple of Christ and the cancer patient. And I have realized that I have always been James. I thank God for giving me Jesus to help me change. To be esteemed in Christ is better than silver or gold!

So what about you? Does your name include being a **disciple of Christ**? How has Christ changed your life?

> **I have been crucified with Christ and**
> **I no longer live, but Christ lives in**
> **me. The life I now live in the body, I**
> **live by faith in the Son of God, who**
> **loved me and gave himself for me.**
>
> **—Galatians 2:20 NIV**

_____

Journal and Prayer

DAY FIFTEEN

**Therefore do not worry about tomorrow,
for tomorrow will worry about itself. Each
day has enough trouble of its own.**

—Matthew 6:34 NIV

**Until we can come face to face with
the deepest, darkest fact of life
without damaging our view of God's
character, we do not yet know Him.**

—Oswald Chambers (utmost.org, July 29)

As my cancer treatments have continued, I could very easily start to dread weekends. The reason for this is that I have chemo every Friday, and I always feel so bad on the weekend. In fact, I usually feel bad until at least Tuesday. There doesn't seem to be anything I can do to overcome this. But Jesus tells us to have a different point of view.

It is important to know that you can count on God while fighting this battle. The proof of this is that God gave us Jesus to overcome our own evil ways, to give us undeserved mercy despite our transgressions. Because God gave us Jesus, **His only son**, to save us, what could He possibly give us that means more to Him than this? Because He has given us Jesus, He has proven that He would give us anything! (Romans 8:32). So we can be absolutely sure of God's love for us! We can absolutely count on God!

So trust Him! Do not concern yourself with the outcome. Trust God, and **give Him** the outcome. Your part is to trust in His goodness and grace so much that you only need to concern yourself with getting through today. For today has enough trouble of its own.

So that is what I have done. I concern myself with only getting through today. I have given the rest to God. I am reminding myself of His goodness and grace. And my bad days have decreased in number!

**You are my strength, I watch for
you; you, God, are my fortress,
my God on whom I can rely.**

—Psalm 59:9–10 (NIV)

———————

Journal and Prayer

DAY SIXTEEN

On the Road to Emmaus

Now that same day two of them were going to a village called Emmaus, about seven miles from Jerusalem. They were talking with each other about everything that had happened. As they talked and discussed these things with each other, Jesus himself came up and walked along with them; but they were kept from recognizing him.

He asked them, "What are you discussing together as you walk along?"

They stood still, their faces downcast. One of them, named Cleopas, asked him, "Are you the only one visiting Jerusalem who does not know the things that have happened there in these days?"

"What things?" he asked.

—Luke 24:13–19a NIV

Let's face it. Being a cancer patient is not easy. From the beginning, even before diagnosis, we have to deal with stress, fear, and maybe pain or discomfort. For me, the biopsy was the worst part. Then there are treatments, pain, side effects, and perhaps loss of income and possibly loss of hair. My beard was one of my casualties. Even after recovery, there can be permanent side effects that can cause great discomfort. My doctor says my lost salivary glands may never return. It can really be, at least, disruptive and, at worst, catastrophic! How do you cope with these unwanted and undeserved problems?

Just as Jesus joined these two disciples as they walked to Emmaus, discussing all the terrible events that had just taken place in their world, Jesus joins us, His children, in our tragedies. He walks with us. He helps us to understand. He comforts us. And He heals us. Just like these disciples, you may not realize that it is He that is walking with you.

As a cancer patient, it is easy to sometimes feel alone or forgotten by God. We may feel like we need to pray, "Lord, do you not see the things that are happening to me?" But our Lord, Jesus Christ, is ever-faithful! He is right beside you, asking, "What things?" He is listening to you with an open heart! Tell Him how you feel. Ask Him to help you. Nothing is impossible for our living Lord! No problem is too big or too small. Bring it all to Jesus in prayer. He is right there with you asking, "What things?"

_____

Journal and Prayer

Day Seventeen

Jesus Changes Water into Wine

On the third day a wedding took place at Cana in Galilee. Jesus' mother was there, and Jesus and his disciples had also been invited to the wedding. When the wine was gone, Jesus' mother said to him, "They have no more wine."

"Woman, why do you involve me?" Jesus replied. "My hour has not yet come."

His mother said to the servants, "Do whatever he tells you."

Nearby stood six stone water jars, the kind used by the Jews for ceremonial washing, each holding from twenty to thirty gallons.

Jesus said to the servants, "Fill the jars with water"; so they filled them to the brim.

Then he told them, "Now draw some out and take it to the master of the banquet."

They did so, and the master of the banquet tasted the water that had been turned into wine. He did not realize where it had come from, though the servants who had drawn the water knew. Then he called the bridegroom aside and said, "Everyone brings out the choice wine first and then the cheaper wine after the guests have had too much to drink; but you have saved the best till now."

What Jesus did here in Cana of Galilee was the first of the signs through which he revealed his glory; and his disciples believed in him.

—John 2:1–11 NIV

The wine jars were empty! The wine was all gone! There was nothing left! They were empty! And soon, the people would be empty as well.

Jesus was just beginning His work as the Messiah. He had yet to perform any miracles. But His mother says to Him, "They have no more wine." You see, she knows who He is. She knows what He can do.

At first, Jesus refuses to do anything to help. He says, "Woman, why do you involve me?" John does not record mother Mary's answer, but we all know what happened next. She gave Him **that look** that only mothers can give - **that look** that we have all seen before. She gave Him **that look** that says, "What in the world are you thinking? Did you not hear what I said? Don't make me tell you again!" And after giving Jesus "**that look**," she tells the servants to do whatever He asks them to do.

Nearby there were some empty ceremonial jars. They, too, were empty. But empty is just what Jesus was looking for. He needed empty jars to fill. He needed empty jars to be able to do His work. Without the empty jars, there would be no miracle.

Have you ever felt empty? It's easy to feel empty with what we are going through as we fight cancer. In fact, life has a way of bringing you to emptiness every once in a while. Our enemy, the devil (the thief), wants you to feel this emptiness. But do not fret if you find yourself feeling empty. As you can see, emptiness is just what Jesus needs!

Because the wine vessels were empty, someone called Jesus to help. Because the ceremonial jars were empty, Jesus had something to fill. Emptiness is the perfect place for Christ to do His work. We all have an emptiness in our hearts that only Christ can fill.

So rejoice in your emptiness! Raise your hands to heaven and give thanks! Ask Jesus to fill your emptiness! And He will fill you to overflowing, completely full! Jesus said,

> **The thief comes only to steal and kill and destroy; I have come that they may have life, and have it to the full. (John 10:10 NIV)**

_____

Journal and Prayer

DAY EIGHTEEN

**Consider it pure joy, my brothers and sisters,
whenever you face trials of many kinds,
because you know that the testing of your
faith produces perseverance. Let perseverance
finish its work so that you may be mature
and complete, not lacking anything.**

—James 1:2–4 NIV

When the world looks at my life and my career, I would imagine that many do not see a man who is successful by worldly standards. There was a time in my life when I did enjoy success in the world. In my late thirties, a friend and colleague at a college where I worked asked me, "Have you always been an overachiever?" But it seems like the closer I have grown to Christ, the less worldly success I have had and the less it mattered. Instead, it has been more important to me to grow closer to God and to become the man that he wants me to be. My measure of success is becoming the person that God wants me to be.

God is the Potter, and we are the clay. He shapes and molds us into the person he wants us to be. But unlike inanimate clay, we have feelings. So being shaped by the Potter can sometimes be a painful process. But it is so worth it! This is the nature of the process of sanctification.

Many people would look at the trials I've had in my life, especially having cancer now, and say, "No, thank you!" It is natural for us to want to live a life that is trouble-free and with the fewest number of trials possible. I feel that way! But at the same time, I am grateful for my trials and for the growth that it has brought to me and the strength it has created in my faith. It has been the trials that have molded and shaped me into the man that God wants me to be. And it has been these trials that have enabled me to serve God and be the disciple of Christ that he wants me to be. This is one of the greatest blessings in my life! I would rather be where I am right now in relationship to God than to have all the money in the world.

Most people in the world make a different choice. In fact, it is interesting to look at people to see the price they have accepted for their soul. That is not to say that anyone who is wealthy or talented has sold their soul to the devil. But the evil one will do whatever he has to do to keep people from coming to Christ and living their lives according to his will in his world. Good news! If this is you, it's not too late! You can turn your life around by accepting Christ today.

The Bible tells us that God also gives wealth to his people. But with God's people, wealth does not replace God. Our God equips his people to do the work for him that they have been called to do. Wealth only becomes evil when it becomes an idol that rivals or replaces God. It is the wealthy who are among God's people that are called to fund his work in this world. Those of us in ministry thank God for providing you for his work.

So do not fret if you do not have success as the world defines it. And do not fret if you have been blessed with great wealth. Keep God first in your life, and seek his leadership in every decision you make (James 1:5). And remember that the trials we have in our life are part of the process of growing us in strength with the Lord. And you, too, will arrive at a point that you can give thanks for the trials in your life. Indeed, they will become for you the Joy of the Lord! You don't want to miss what God has for you!

**Blessed is the one who perseveres under
trial because, having stood the test, that**

**person will receive the crown of life that the
Lord has promised to those who love him.**

—James 1:12 NIV

_____

Journal and Prayer

DAY NINETEEN

**Praise be to the God and Father of
our Lord Jesus Christ, the Father of
compassion and the God of all comfort.**

—1 Corinthians 1:3 NIV

Cancer is a disease that can knock you down to your knees. But believe it or not, there is no better place to be, no better place from which to reach out to God.

I know that may sound crazy! But our God is the God of all comfort. He knows your pains and will help you as you work to overcome. If you will bathe yourself daily in God's Word, it will put you on the right path. Our objective is to become one with Christ and one with the Father. Pray whenever you have a moment. Seek the face of the Lord! And study His Word!

Develop a habit of prayer. Prayer gives you breakthrough power! I pray, for example, whenever the Holy Spirit moves me. I pray if I have trouble sleeping. And I pray during my entire radiation treatment. Here's a new one for me. After getting the idea from a pastor friend, I have decided to pray at 6:10 p.m. each day. The time comes from Ephesians 6:10, but you can use whatever verse the Spirit leads you to.

Finally, be strong in the Lord and in his mighty power. (Ephesians 6:10 NIV)

This doesn't have to be permanent, but for a season, it will help me to remember to pray. And it helps me to internalize God's promises.

Our God created all things! With Him, all things are possible! He raises people from death. He restores life! Our Lord is mighty indeed! We don't need a smaller view of our problems. We need a bigger view of our God! There is nothing outside of the reach of God! He who has raised people from the dead can also heal disease!

But I will sing of your strength, in the morning I will sing of your love; for you are my fortress, my refuge in times of trouble. (Psalm 59:16 NIV)

Focus your attention not on the fight but on what is beyond the fight. We are more than conquerors! Visualize being well and feeling good again. I have now reached the midpoint of my treatments, and I am celebrating! Celebrate your milestones! Most importantly, remember that God brings all of His strength and power to you if you ask Him. Without Him, you may be helpless. But with Him, all things are possible! How big do you see our God?

Finally, you need to know Christ Jesus. He is the best way to know our Father (John 14:8–10). The Son is the radiance of God's glory (Hebrews 1:3). Jesus is the way.

But he was pierced for our transgressions, he was crushed for our iniquities; the punishment that brought us peace was on him, and by his wounds we are healed. (Isaiah 53:5 NIV)

Remember, you are getting closer to being well again every day! But you do have to go through your treatments to get there. God is blessing you along the way! Lean into our Lord and Savior! Learn about how great our God is by spending time in His Word and time in prayer. Sing a new song to the Lord and receive His Blessings!

Journal and Prayer

DAY TWENTY

**The strong spirit of a man sustains him
in bodily pain or trouble, but a weak and
broken spirit who can raise up or bear?**

—Proverbs 18:14 AMPC

As you grow in strength in the Lord, the evil one will bring trouble to you to try to unseat your faith. But through the trial, you will find your faith; you will know just how strong your faith is. The trial is evidence that your faith is worthy of note by the evil one. You are a child of faith!

But remember that Jesus accomplished the resurrection for our salvation only after dying on the cross. So remain undaunted! Your faith will power you through this trial! And you must go through—this is the only way. God is with you, and He will help you to power through!

I can do all this through him who gives me strength. (Philippians 4:13 NIV)

You cannot know how strong your faith is without the trial. It is the trial that shows you the measure of your faith. You should know that you will win this battle because you know Christ and know His strength is in you. Rejoice in this constantly, and you will overcome every battle! And if you do not think that you are there yet, ask God to help you with your faith, for He is a God who gives generously!

In conclusion, be strong in the Lord! Be empowered through your union with Him and draw your strength from Him—that strength which His boundless might provides (Ephesians 6:10 AMPC).

> **[For my determined purpose is] that I may know Him [that I may progressively become more deeply and intimately acquainted with Him, perceiving and recognizing and understanding the wonders of His Person more strongly and more clearly], and that I may in that same way come to know the power outflowing from His resurrection [which it exerts over believers], and that I may so share His sufferings as to be continually transformed [in spirit into His likeness even] to His death. (Philippians 3:10 AMPC)**

You have what it takes in Christ to win this battle! God is faithful! He is with you and is faithful to see you through your trial!

> **Give thanks in all circumstances; for this is God's will for you in Christ Jesus. (1 Thessalonians 5:18 NIV)**

Additional thoughts:

- Because of my cancer, I hear new things in God's Word that I have never heard before.
- Cancer is never a death sentence, no matter how fatal for those who are in Christ.
- I am humbled by how many people are praying for me. Some of them are people whom I don't even know!

Journal and Prayer

DAY TWENTY-ONE

**Therefore God exalted him to the highest
place and gave him the name that is above
every name, that at the name of Jesus
every knee should bow, in heaven and
on earth and under the earth, and every
tongue acknowledge that Jesus Christ is
Lord, to the glory of God the Father.**

—Philippians 2:9–11 NIV

There's an older guy at work, whom I really like, who constantly called me by a different name (despite wearing a name tag). I have never corrected him because I like him and do not want him to feel bad or embarrassed. I gladly answer to the name he has given me.

Our name is a significant part of our personal identity. Our name is ours. For this reason, people are often quick to correct when another person gets their name wrong. We feel compelled to stand up for who we are. After all, we have a right to what is ours; we have a right to ourselves. Or do we?

This right to ourselves is what drives a major part of the human psyche that always asks, "What about me?" It is the source of our desire to demand to be treated right. It is the root of selfishness. But God wants us to give up this selfishness and give ourselves completely to Him.

God is a God of justice. He knows when you are being mistreated and when you are being treated unfairly. That is not to say that because God is a God of justice, you should not stand up for yourself. But the first place to start is in prayer, asking the Holy Spirit to lead you.

There are two terrific examples of people who lived their lives this way. The most prominent is Jesus Christ Himself, who being fully God and fully man, did not count His divinity as something to be used to have His way. Instead, He submitted Himself to God and made Himself a servant to all, even to the point of submitting Himself to death on the cross. And doing so, He achieved forgiveness for all mankind (Philippians 2:5–11).

The other example is Martin Luther King Jr. Dr. King said, "The end of life is not to be happy, nor to achieve pleasure and avoid pain, but to do the will of God, come what may." We should all strive to live this way.

In Jesus's day, people named their children for what they expected them to become. God named His Son Jesus, which means Savior. If you want God to fix the peripheral problems in your life, then accept His gift of Christ to fix the primary problem in your life of sin. Otherwise, you really have no right to expect anything.

Journal and Prayer

Day Twenty-Two

Whoever dwells in the shelter of the Most High will rest in the shadow of the Almighty.

I will say of the Lord, "He is my refuge and my fortress, my God, in whom I trust."

Surely he will save you from the fowler's snare and from the deadly pestilence.

He will cover you with his feathers, and under his wings you will find refuge;

his faithfulness will be your shield and rampart.

You will not fear the terror of night, nor the arrow that flies by day.

—Psalm 91:1–5 NIV

I heard about a little girl who was born with a severe allergy to eggs. It was so severe that even touching an egg could send her to the hospital. As a little girl, she learned to always ask whether something contained eggs before touching it. At birthday parties, she would ask,

"Does the cake have eggs in it?"

"Does the ice cream have eggs in it?"

"Does the Kool-Aid have eggs in it?"

And she would resolve herself to have only the Kool-Aid. Starting when she was three years old, she would tell everyone, "When I turn six, I will be able to eat eggs." She said this with certainty, calling it out from the Lord and believing that God would deliver her. And when she was six years old, she was no longer allergic to eggs!

This little girl grew up in a godly family. Her parents and grandparents are devout Christians. So she saw them living in the shelter of the Lord and learned early on who God is and about His faithfulness.

We must also learn who God is and come to Him as this small child did, expecting to see the deliverance of our faithful God. It doesn't matter what kind of family you grew up in. If you are reading this, God is calling you to **His** family. He wants you to know who He is, just as the little girl knows who He is. There's a place for you to rest in His shadow.

Journal and Prayer

Day Twenty-Three

Hezekiah's Illness

In those days Hezekiah became ill and was at the point of death. The prophet Isaiah son of Amoz went to him and said, "This is what the Lord says: Put your house in order, because you are going to die; you will not recover."

Hezekiah turned his face to the wall and prayed to the Lord, "Remember, Lord, how I have walked before you faithfully and with wholehearted devotion and have done what is good in your eyes." And Hezekiah wept bitterly.

—2 Kings 20:1–3 NIV

A colleague at work, whom I have been praying for, lost his battle with cancer this week. This man was a top performer and very wealthy. Yet his performance and wealth did not save him. And as I prayed for him, God told me that he wanted his heart. I never saw my colleague turn his heart to God. Instead, he spent tens of thousands of dollars on medicines to try and save his own life.

Jesus told us it is easier for a camel to get through the eye of a needle than for a wealthy man to make it into heaven. This is not because being wealthy is sinful or necessarily a bad thing, but it is because wealth and position can take the place of God. It becomes an idol in our lives. Often, wealth or position can make you believe that you do not need God. Many of the wealthy either do not fully submit to God (keeping their wealth first in importance) or ignore Him completely.

In this passage, Hezekiah prays to the Lord and pleads his case, reminding the Lord of how much he loves Him and how devoted he has been. God decides to heal Hezekiah. The passage tells us,

> **Before Isaiah had left the middle court, the word of the Lord came to him: "Go back and tell Hezekiah, the ruler of my people, 'This is what the Lord, the God of your father David, says: I have heard your prayer and seen your tears; I will heal you.**

All of Hezekiah's wealth and position could not save him. But his heart for God could. He was healed when he set aside his wealth and position and got down on his knees.

We are called to live our lives for God. Oswald Chambers tells us in *My Utmost for His Highest* (December 2) that we are called to live in such perfect relationship with God that our lives produce a yearning for God in the lives of others, not admiration for ourselves. God's purpose is not to perfect us to make us trophies for His showcase but rather to get us to the place where He can use us for His work and glory. This should be our primary objective in life (Oswald Chambers, Utmost.org, December 2). What would happen to this world if we all lived our lives this way?

God Almighty, Creator of all things, would like to have a personal relationship with you. He wants your heart. He loves you, and He wants you to love Him. It is when you put him first in your life that He can begin to use you to do wonderful things in this world. My colleague missed out on these things. It is my prayer that you will not.

Let the morning bring me word of your unfailing love, for I have put my trust in you. Show me the way I should go, for to you I entrust my life. (Psalm 143:8 NIV)

As you grow closer to God, you too will find that you dwell in the shelter of the Most High. And whoever dwells in the shelter of the Most High will rest in the shadow of the Almighty. He will be your refuge and shelter. You will find in Him the God whom you can trust.

_____

Journal and Prayer

DAY TWENTY-FOUR

**For I resolved to know nothing
while I was with you except Jesus
Christ and him crucified.**

—Corinthians 2:2 NIV

Fighting cancer is not for the faint of heart! It takes more strength than we can muster on our own. That's why we need God so much to help us make it through to the end. When Christ chose the apostle Paul to be His champion to bring the Gospel to the Gentiles, Paul, who was then called Saul, was a very strong character. But he was probably the greatest enemy that Christians had. Saul killed more Christians than anyone else before he met Christ on the road to Damascus. Yet he became one of the most influential apostles of Christ.

The apostle Paul **met** the **risen Christ** on the road to Damascus. He talked to Him. More than that, he had a conversation with Him. And Christ had blinded him to get his attention. As a result, Paul, who had formerly been known as Saul, became a new man, bringing the Gospel to most of the world and writing two-thirds of the New Testament in the Bible. Yet despite meeting Christ in person, in our scripture today, Paul tells us that his most important objective is to know Jesus Christ better.

Before Paul did anything for the Lord, he was blinded. It took being blind and meeting the risen Christ to give Paul the drive to serve. It often takes something dramatic in our lives for God to get our attention and to put us on a new path for Him. What is God giving you through your illness? Is He planting a new drive, new call, new mission in your life? Ask Him to show you the way! Commit yourself to become the person God wants you—needs you—to be for Him.

Our God is the one who can turn all things into good! Paul had to be blinded before he was willing to listen to Christ. But once he did, he became one of the most useful people to ever be used by God. Ask God what you can do for Him. Ask Him to fill you with His Holy Spirit and to guide you day by day. Whether He wants you to lead your family to Christ or to work in an important ministry, or whatever His plan is for you, I promise you that you will find fulfillment in pursuing it.

This is where you will find the strength to be thankful even now. It is in having a purpose that is greater than being sick that you will find that strength. Perhaps having cancer is leading you to that greater purpose! Lean into our all-loving God!

**Give thanks in all circumstances; for this
is God's will for you in Christ Jesus.**

—1 Thessalonians 5:18 NIV

_____

Journal and Prayer

DAY TWENTY-FIVE

"The days are coming," declares the Sovereign Lord, "when I will send a famine through the land—not a famine of food or a thirst for water, but a famine of hearing the words of the Lord.

—Amos 8:11 NIV

But mark this: There will be terrible times in the last days. People will be lovers of themselves, lovers of money, boastful, proud, abusive, disobedient to their parents, ungrateful, unholy, without love, unforgiving, slanderous, without self-control, brutal, not lovers of the good, treacherous, rash, conceited, lovers of pleasure rather than lovers of God—having a form of godliness but denying its power. Have nothing to do with such people.

—2 Timothy 3:1–5 NIV

Do you know people like this? Are you like this? It is easy to see that this scripture describes the world we live in today. This is the way the world today teaches us to live, and most people live their lives this

66

way. Jesus calls us to live our lives a different way. We are called to be disciples of Christ.

> **Then he said to them all: "Whoever wants to be my disciple must deny themselves and take up their cross daily and follow me." (Luke 9:23 NIV)**

It greatly saddens me to see how our churches have set up a throne of politics in the sanctuary next to the throne of God. And many denominations are now choosing a policy based on politics instead of the Word of God. This is an abomination! We cannot expect God's blessings as long as we insult Him in this way! In fact, He would be completely justified in punishing those who do this. But the world is telling us that this is the way to go. And many are listening. No matter what we feel, if what we feel disagrees with God's Word, God's Word is still always right. As long as we keep living by our feelings and don't confront the lies of the evil one, the devil will always have the upper hand.

> **Then from his mouth the serpent spewed water like a river, to overtake the woman and sweep her away with the torrent. (Revelation 12:15 NIV)**

In this prophetic scripture, the water is the evil one's word, his religion, and the woman is the church. Satan wants to turn you from God's Word to his way of thinking. So if this is you who has turned your back on the Word of God, repent! Return to the Word of God! And as the apostle Paul wrote,

> **Follow my example, as I follow the example of Christ. (1 Corinthians 11:1 NIV)**

Remember: out of the abundance of the heart, the mouth speaks (Matthew 12:34). So fill your heart with the Word of God. Ignore the evening news and the messages that the world is giving you. Ask God to fill you with His Holy Spirit and Word. Study the Word of God and rid yourself of any pastor or church that teaches anything other than the Word of God.

_____

Journal and Prayer

Day Twenty-Six

**In your relationships with one another,
have the same mindset as Christ Jesus.**

—Philippians 2:5 NIV

**Oh, what a happy soul I am, although I cannot
see! I am resolved that in this world Contented
I will be. How many blessings I enjoy That
other people don't, To weep and sigh because
I'm blind I cannot, and I won't!**

This is the first poem of Fanny Crosby, who was born in 1820. She wrote this poem when she was eight years old. Fanny was born with sight. When she was six weeks old, she contracted a fever. Her family doctor was out of town, and she was treated instead by someone who was pretending to be a doctor. He put a mustard paste on her eyes, and as a result, she lost her sight. Fanny wrote more than nine thousand hymns, and they are used by every denomination. She had written so many hymns that she used a *pen name* on some of them she wrote so that her name would not appear in hymnals so much.

Fanny never felt sorry for herself. A well-meaning pastor once said to her, "You have so many gifts and talents. It's a shame that God did not give you your sight." Fanny did not agree "because when I get to heaven," she said, "the first face that shall ever gladden my sight will be that of my Savior." I think one of the biggest challenges we have is to not feel sorry for ourselves. Our scripture today tells us to have the same mindset as Christ. Christ came to the Earth knowing all things and what He faced. In the garden of Gethsemane, He did pray to God and asked to not have to go through it. But He capped off His prayer by saying, "Not my will, but your will be done." I think the key to not feeling sorry for yourself is simply trusting in God. When you understand the fullness of God's mercy and grace as found in Jesus Christ, when you understand that God takes all things and makes them work for your good, it gives you a certain confidence that can only be found in the life of the Savior and in trusting our Almighty God.

So whatever you might be facing, whatever you might be going through, God's got this! You can trust the one who loves you so much that He gave you His only son. You can trust the one who went to the cross for you! He's got this, and so do you! So start looking for and expecting the blessings that God has in store for you.

―――――――――――

Journal and Prayer

DAY TWENTY-SEVEN

**Jesus looked at them and said, "With
man this is impossible, but with
God all things are possible."**

—Matthew 19:26 NIV

I enjoy listening to Joyce Meyer. She tells it like it is. In one of her recent messages, Joyce said this, "Pray, say, and do." She says to kneel before the throne of God and make your requests known. In your everyday life, let your words match your requests by prayer as if it is happening and coming true now. Expect a positive outcome from your prayer, knowing that your Father, who knows all things, would not give you something that would do you harm. Then align your actions with your requests, ignoring the negative thoughts thrown at you by the evil one and taking actions based on your positive expectation. "Pray, say, and do."

You have to trust and hold on. God's timing is perfect, and He always honors His promises. Max Lucado says, "Don't tell God how big your storm is. Tell your storm how big your God is." Wrap your mind around who God is!

**For the Lord your God is God of gods and
Lord of lords, the great God, mighty and awe-**

71

some, who shows no partiality and accepts no bribes. (Deuteronomy 10:17 NIV)

Now try to understand His immense strength and power and goodness!

Oh, magnify the Lord with me, And let us exalt His name together. (Psalm 34:3 NKJV)

And remember His promises to you and to all who call Him "Abba!"

And we know that in all things God works for the good of those who love him, who have been called according to his purpose. (Romans 8:28 NIV)

If you are reading this, you are one of those called by God! He is greater than you can imagine! He is much greater than any diagnosis! He is greater than your storm! Let us magnify the name of the Lord!

_____

Journal and Prayer

DAY TWENTY-EIGHT

God's Revelation to Elijah

Then He said, "Go out, and stand on the mountain before the Lord." And behold, the Lord passed by, and a great and strong wind tore into the mountains and broke the rocks in pieces before the Lord, but the Lord was not in the wind; and after the wind an earthquake, but the Lord was not in the earthquake; and after the earthquake a fire, but the Lord was not in the fire; and after the fire a still small voice. So it was, when Elijah heard it, that he wrapped his face in his mantle and went out and stood in the entrance of the cave. Suddenly a voice came to him, and said, "What are you doing here, Elijah?"

—1 Kings 19:11–13 NKJV

How good are you at hearing from God? Most people only live in the five senses (sight, smell, touch, etc.). But as a Christian, God will interact with you in your spirit. You receive this spirit when you are born again. Jesus tells us about this in John 3:

Jesus answered, "Very truly I tell you, no one can enter the kingdom of God unless they are born of water and the Spirit. Flesh gives birth to flesh, but the Spirit gives birth to spirit. (John 3:5–6 NIV)

So when you receive the Holy Spirit, your spirit is born within you. Along with accepting Christ, this is one of the keys to living in the kingdom of God on earth. God tells us in Ezekiel,

I will give you a new heart and put a new spirit in you; I will remove from you your heart of stone and give you a heart of flesh. (Ezekiel 36:26 NIV)

Like your muscles and your mind, you must develop your spirit by using it. You develop your spirit as you develop your faith.

To develop your spirit is to become tuned into it. Worship, prayer, Bible study, spending time with other believers, and time spent serving God will help your spirit to become a powerful resource within you and help you to discover and fulfill the call God has on your life as one of His children. As you develop your spirit more fully, you become more tuned into God and better able to discern His voice.

This is essential to any Christian! You want to be more than just a cultural Christian. You want to be filled and led by the Holy Spirit and equipped to do His work. Let me show you why. When I was in seminary, the denomination of which I am a member was holding its International Conference in a nearby city. My seminary had invited students to attend a luncheon they were holding there on Tuesday. Normally on Tuesdays, I would attend a men's breakfast meeting and then return home to study for the rest of the day. But since I wanted to attend the luncheon, I decided to study at a local doughnut shop instead and save twenty minutes from my drive to the luncheon. After I sat down with my coffee and doughnuts to study, I felt the Spirit of the Lord speaking to me. He said, "Buy two doughnuts and a cup of coffee, and take them to a man at a place that I will show you. Tell him to stay in faith and that God is working things out for him."

In my spirit, God showed me a downtown location with a bridge in the background. I did as the Spirit told me and left immediately on my journey. As I arrived in the downtown area of the city, I began to recognize the location from the image given to me in my mind's eye by the Holy Spirit. There was a single man standing on the corner selling newspapers. I pulled in. As I exited the car, carrying the doughnuts and coffee, the man beamed with a big smile. I said to him, "You're not going to believe this, but God told me to bring these doughnuts to you and to give you a message. He says to stay in faith and that He is working things out for you." As I handed him the coffee and doughnuts, he said, "Yes, I would believe that!" I stayed on the corner that morning and talked to him until it was time to leave for my luncheon. I am glad I was able to be used by God for His purposes. I think you can see how important it is to develop your spirit so you can be used by God for His purposes. I was greatly blessed in being able to serve God that day. And I know the man on the corner really needed that Word from God. So be diligent in developing your spiritual life with God. There's no substitute for being intimate with God through your own spirit.

In closing, I leave you with this prayer from the apostle Paul:

> **I pray that out of his glorious riches he may strengthen you with power through his Spirit in your inner being, so that Christ may dwell in your hearts through faith. And I pray that you, being rooted and established in love, may have power, together with all the Lord's holy people, to grasp how wide and long and high and deep is the love of Christ, and to know this love that surpasses knowledge—that you may be filled to the measure of all the fullness of God. (Ephesians 3:16–19 NI)**
>
> **Amen!**

Journal and Prayer

Day Twenty-Nine

The Time Is Now

**Let the morning bring me word of
your unfailing love, for I have put my
trust in you. Show me the way I should
go, for to you I entrust my life.**

—Psalm 143:8 NIV

Twenty years ago, I was working for a "dot-com," a start-up company whose business model involved using this new technology called the Internet to bring products and services to the public. It was an exciting time, and we all felt that if we worked hard and created a useful product, we would become wealthy and successful. Our motto was, "The time is now!"

This is a good motto for those of us who have cancer too. The time is now for us to take steps to fight the disease in our bodies. The time is now to focus on what and who is really important in our lives. The time is now to get our lives in order. And **the time is now** to grow in Christ and lean into the grace and love of our all-powerful God!

In Christ alone, we find hope. His work while He walked this earth was to teach us about our Father. He did this by giving us parables, defying the religious zealots, and healing the sick. Yes, Jesus heals the sick for, by His stripes, we are healed! He came for you and me!

So let the living Lord hear your prayer that in His faithfulness and righteousness, He may come to your aid. Let the morning bring you the word of His unfailing love, for you have put your trust in Him! He will show you the way! You can trust Him with your very life!

The Lord says to you,

> **I have summoned you by name; you are mine.**
>
> **When you pass through the waters, I will be with you; and when you pass through the rivers, they will not sweep over you. When you walk through the fire, you will not be burned; the flames will not set you ablaze.**
>
> **For I am the Lord your God, the Holy One of Israel, your Savior; I give Egypt for your ransom, Cush and Seba in your stead. (Isaiah 43:1b–3 NIV)**
> **Glory Just Around the Corner**
>
> **Friends, when life gets really difficult, don't jump to the conclusion that God isn't on the job. Instead, be glad that you are in the very thick of what Christ experienced. This is a spiritual refining process, with glory just around the corner. (1 Peter 4:12–13 MSG)**

The time is now! Forget the past. Leave your future in God's hands. Focus on now with God!

———————

Journal and Prayer

DAY THIRTY

But when he, the Spirit of truth, comes, he will guide you into all the truth. He will not speak on his own; he will speak only what he hears, and he will tell you what is yet to come.

—John 16:13 NIV

Two natures live within your breast.
The one is foul, the one is blessed.
The one you love, the one you hate,
The one you feed will dominate!

—Dr. David Jeremiah

In 1953, Christian Broadcasting Network founder, Pat Robertson, was living in New York with his wife and three kids when God told him to "sell what you have, give to the poor, and come follow me." Pat sold all of his furniture, asked a friend to give the proceeds to the poor, and moved with his wife and three children to Tidewater, Virginia, with a DeSoto (car) and $70 in his pocket. God then told him to buy a TV station, and Pat didn't even own a television! How many millions of people have been blessed through CBN?

Abiding in Christ is not for those of little faith! But if you can develop your faith to this level, you can be guided by God in all that you do. Imagine being led by the one who knows ALL things, who knows the beginning before the end! Pat Robertson's life shows you what a life lived this way is like. His life shows the incredible fruit that comes with abiding in Christ.

To abide in Christ is to obey Him. In *My Utmost for His Highest*, Oswald Chambers wrote, "If I obey Jesus Christ, the redemption of God will flow through me to the lives of others, because behind the deed of obedience is the reality of Almighty God" (Utmost.org, November 2). There is no better way to live your life and no better way to fulfill the will of God for your life. Just imagine how many lives God can bless through you if you will abide in Him!

Abiding in Christ is accomplished in this way:

- Spend the first part of each day with God in the study of His Word and prayer. Ask, "What are the things you want me to do today?" Don't end your morning time with the Lord until He dismisses you.
- Journal daily—write out your questions for Christ and what the Lord is speaking to you in your spirit.
- Hear from God—Most people only live in the five senses (sight, smell, touch, etc.). But God will interact with you in your spirit. Follow His leading, and you will be amazed by where He leads you.
- Step into obedience, bearing fruit by doing the work God asks you to do.
- Pray throughout the day. Commune with God. Come before Him in all you do, living in His loving presence (1 Thessalonians 5:17).

You hear from God through the Holy Spirit. He speaks to you in your spirit that was born in you when you accepted Christ. If you're not hearing from God, ask God to show you the gap.

The Spirit of the Lord will come
powerfully upon you, and you will

**prophesy with them; and you will be
changed into a different person.**

—1 Samuel 10:6 NIV

_____

Journal and Prayer

DAY THIRTY-ONE

**Suddenly a sound like the blowing of a
violent wind came from heaven and filled the
whole house where they were sitting. They
saw what seemed to be tongues of fire that
separated and came to rest on each of them.
All of them were filled with the Holy Spirit.**

—Acts 2:2–4 NIV

For our "God is a consuming fire."

—Hebrews 12:29 NIV

In biblical times before Jesus Christ, the Jewish people would bring
a dove, lamb, bull, or some other unblemished animal to be sacrificed at the temple as an atonement for their sins. The priest would
inspect the gift of sacrifice, assuring that it was unblemished. Then
once accepted, the sacrifice would be put on the fire. The aroma of
their sacrifice burning was pleasing to God, and God would forgive
their sins.

When Jesus Christ, the Lamb of God, died for our sins, no
more animal sacrifices were needed. Our bodies became God's temple, and the perfect, unblemished Lamb of God was sacrificed for us

once and for all. Praise God! For the sacrificed and resurrected Christ lives in you and me.

This sacrifice is still made with fire. For many of us, it is the fire in our lives that brings us to Christ to begin with. It is the fire in our lives that drives us to our knees to seek God and to give our lives fully to His will. It is the fire in our lives that sanctifies us and helps us to become the people that God wants us to be. It is the fire in our lives that ignites our hearts and drives us to do the work of Almighty God! Once we understand this, we can begin to be thankful for the fires in our lives. Fire that is out of control is devastating. But fire that is purposeful and in control can accomplish great things!

After Christ's sacrifice, the apostles were not anointed for the work they were chosen to do until they were baptized by the fire of the Holy Spirit. And so it is with you. This cancer is your fire. You are now more empowered to grow in Christ and do the work He has prepared for you to do. Let the Spirit lead you!

So this cancer, this fire in your life, is a fire that enhances the sacrifice of Jesus Christ. It is the fire that purifies your heart and your mind. It is the fire that cleanses you of sin. It is the fire that ignites you for God's work.

> **Jesus said, "If you hold to my teaching, you**
> **are really my disciples. Then you will know**
> **the truth, and the truth will set you free."**
>
> **—John 8:31–32 NIV**

Journal and Prayer

CLOSING

**Yet it was the Lord's will to crush him and
cause him to suffer, and though the Lord
makes his life an offering for sin, he will see
his offspring and prolong his days, and the
will of the Lord will prosper in his hand.**

—Isaiah 53:10 NIV

God did not crucify Jesus, man did. But God allowed it to fulfill His
good, divine will to save mankind. If God has allowed cancer in your
life, it is for His good purpose. Maybe you do not belong to Him,
and He wants you. Maybe He wants you to grow closer to Him.
Maybe He has some special work for you to do.

Is the will of the Lord prospering in your hands? Christ has a
place for you in His kingdom, and He has work for you to do that
you have been uniquely equipped to do.

**So Christ himself gave the apostles, the proph-
ets, the evangelists, the pastors and teachers, to
equip his people for works of service, so that
the body of Christ may be built up until we
all reach unity in the faith and in the knowl-
edge of the Son of God and become mature,**

**attaining to the whole measure of the fullness
of Christ. (Ephesians 4:11–13 NIV)**

Prayerfully find your place and pursue it, fulfilling God's call on your life. Christ is counting on you, and you can count on Christ.

**For God's gifts and his call are irrevocable.
(Romans 11:29 NIV)**

I had a PET scan on Monday and found out this week that they did not see any cancer cells in my body. Hallelujah! However, my doctor did not say that I was cancer-free. Instead, the doctor declared that I was in remission. That's okay; I'll take it! Whatever it is, I have given it to God, and I praise Him for it! I trust Him to turn all things into good as He has promised.

**And we know that in all things God works
for the good of those who love him, who have
been called according to his purpose. (Romans
8:28 NIV)**

I could not have written this book of devotions without going through my journey with cancer. It is my prayer that this book of devotions has blessed you as much as it has blessed me. After all, in giving these devotions to me, the Holy Spirit was nurturing my spirit and bringing healing to my soul. He has given me strength to endure and undaunted faith to face any outcome, fully trusting in the grace and love and goodness of God as found in Jesus Christ. It is my prayer that you have experienced these same gifts from God!

The truth is, I did not know whether I would be healed in this life or the next. Sometimes we do not experience healing until we go to live with God. But I trusted my Savior either way. I still have a few battles to fight as I work to overcome the impact on my body of this disease. But God is with me in these battles as well. He will generously provide for me to eliminate the things that he wants to be eliminated and to live with the things he wants me to keep. Praise

God! His Grace is enough! And he will do the same for you. He is worthy of your trust!

> **But he said to me, "My grace is sufficient for you, for my power is made perfect in weakness." Therefore I will boast all the more gladly about my weaknesses, so that Christ's power may rest on me. (2 Corinthians 12:9 NIV)**

Once when Christ was speaking to a large multitude of people, the time arrived to have a meal. Our Savior asked His disciples, "What do you think it will take to feed all these people?" One of the disciples thought it would take a year's wages. But all they found among the people was a little boy who had a few fish and a few loaves of bread. And with this, they fed everyone!

> **When they had all had enough to eat, he said to his disciples, "Gather the pieces that are left over. Let nothing be wasted." ¹So they gathered them and filled twelve baskets with the pieces of the five barley loaves left over by those who had eaten. (John 6:12–13 NIV)**

Gather the pieces of your life, and you will be amazed by what Christ can do with them! Now may the Lord of peace bless you and keep you; may He make His face shine upon you. And may He give you His peace and healing as only He can! **Amen** and **amen!**

ABOUT THE AUTHOR

In writing, Jamie Byrd shares what the Holy Spirit is teaching and sharing with him. As a Christian since childhood, he has navigated the ups and downs of life and faith, finally realizing that Christ truly is the way, the truth, and the life. For Jamie, writing is an act of worship, study, and discipleship. It is a means to grow closer to Christ, to prayerfully learn wisdom from the Lord, and to share the Gospel with the world. He lives in Florida with his wife, Barb, and his Labrador retriever, Katie.